The Diverticulitis Diet Cookbook For Seniors

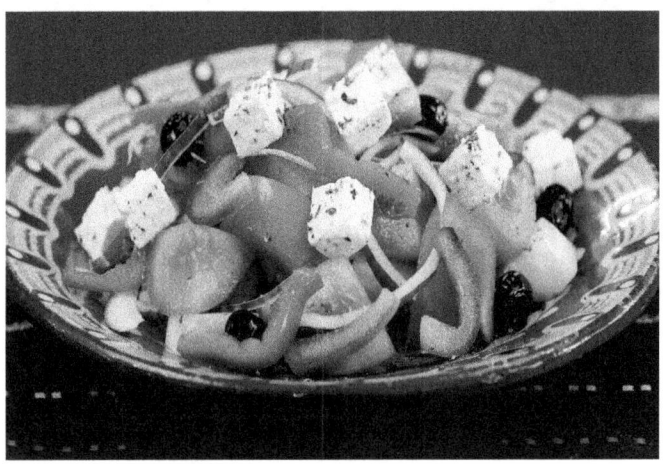

A Comprehensive Guide to Managing Diverticulitis Symptoms and Promoting Digestive Health

Cassy Jane

COPYRIGHT PAGE

Copyright © 2024 By Cassy Jane

All rights reserved. No part of this publication may be reproduced, distributed, or transmitted in any form or by any means, including photocopying, recording, or other electronic or mechanical methods, without the prior written permission of the copyright owner.

This work is protected by copyright law and other international intellectual property laws. Any unauthorized reproduction, distribution, or transmission of this work is strictly prohibited.

ACKNOWLEDGMENT

Firstly, I want to thank God from the bottom of my heart for directing me as I created this senior diverticulitis illness cookbook. I have always found strength and direction in your heavenly presence and inspiration.

I also want to express my gratitude to God for his grace and the testimonials of the patients who have valiantly fought against this difficult illness. Your fortitude, bravery, and openness to sharing your stories have been crucial in molding this cookbook and offering insightful advice to anyone traveling a similar path.

I want to express my sincere gratitude to the reader who has bought this book for their support and faith in me. I sincerely hope that the recipes and information found within these pages will help you or your loved ones who are suffering with diverticulitis feel better, nourished, and healed.

Finally, I'd like to introduce myself as this cookbook's author, Cassy Jane. Developing this resource for anyone looking to enhance their health and wellbeing through thoughtful and nourishing cooking has been a privilege and an honor.

We are grateful to everyone who helped make this cookbook a reality. I think it will be a source of empowerment and optimism for anyone dealing with diverticulitis. Continue to be healthy, powerful, and to cook with love

With appreciation,
Cassy Jane

BOOK NAVIGATING GUIDE

1. Introduction: - To learn about the author's inspiration and motivation for writing this cookbook, read the acknowledgements.

- Learn about the author, Cassy Jane, and her dedication to offering wholesome recipes to those who suffer from diverticulitis.

2. Understanding Diverticulitis: - Acquire knowledge about the signs, causes, and dietary guidelines associated with diverticulitis.

- Learn from the stories and testimonies of others who have struggled with this illness.

3. Recipe Section: - Choose from a selection of delectable and simple meals created especially for elderly people suffering from diverticulitis.

- Every recipe is designed to be easy on the stomach while still offering vital nutrients for good health.

4. Getting Around the Recipes: - For convenience, the recipes are divided into categories according to the kinds of meals (breakfast, lunch, supper, and snacks).

- Look for recipe comments that specify any dietary adjustments or concerns that should be made for those who have diverticulitis.

5. Cooking Techniques and Advice: - To support a diverticulitis-friendly diet, find useful advice on item replacements, cooking techniques, and portion control.

- Find strategies to improve textures and flavors without sacrificing the health of your digestive system.

6. Meal Planning and Preparation: - Make pleasant, well-balanced meal plans that follow the nutritional guidelines for diverticulitis by using the meal planning guide.

- For convenience and time savings, learn how to prepare meals ahead of time and store leftovers safely.

7. Conclusion: - Contemplate how vital it is to cook with love and intention in order to nourish the body and the soul.

- Accept the path towards improved health and wellbeing by engaging in self-care and mindful eating.

By using this guide, readers can easily navigate the Diverticulitis Disease Cookbook for Seniors, making wise decisions and savoring satisfying meals that promote their journey toward better health.

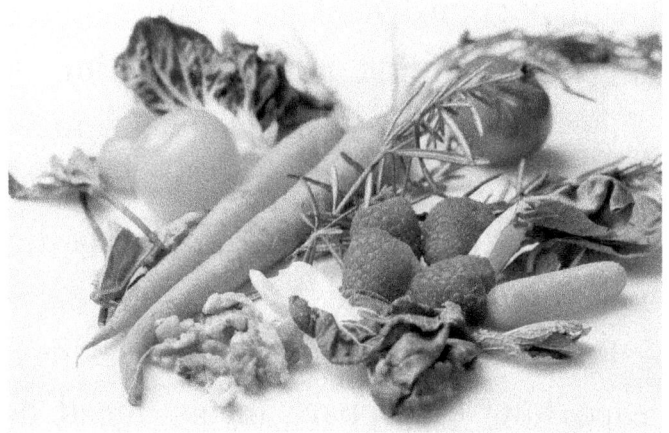

Table of contents

ACKNOWLEDGMENT	4
BOOK NAVIGATING GUIDE	6
INTRODUCTION	11
CHAPTER 1	17
FOODS TO EAT AND AVOID	17
Benefits of following a Diverticulitis Diet	22
CHAPTER 2	27
HOW TO FOLLOW A DIVERTICULITIS DIET	27
SHOPPING INGREDIENTS	30
Diverticulitis Disease Complications	34
CHAPTER 1	39
MEAL PLANNING	39
Benefits of Proper Meal Planning	42
SIMPLE MEAL PLAN	45
CHAPTER 4	50
BREAKFAST RECIPES	50
LUNCH RECIPES	57
DINNER RECIPES	64
SNACKS RECIPES	71
CONCLUSION	77

INTRODUCTION

𝓐 common digestive disorder that mostly affects the large intestine of the colon is diverticulitis. It happens when tiny pouches known as diverticula grow in the colon's lining and get infected or inflammatory. Numerous symptoms, such as bloating, abdominal pain, altered bowel habits, and in more serious situations, problems including abscesses or perforations, may result from this.

Diverticulitis can be classified into two primary categories: **simple and complex.** While difficult diverticulitis comprises more severe symptoms and possible problems such abscess formation, colon perforation, or fistulas, uncomplicated diverticulitis is defined as inflammation of the diverticula without any serious complications.

Diverticulitis's precise etiology is unknown, however a number of variables, such as age, genetics, nutrition, and lifestyle, are thought to be involved. Age is one of the main risk factors for diverticulitis, with people over 40 having a higher prevalence of the illness. Given that certain individuals may be genetically predisposed to having diverticula in the colon, genetics may potentially be involved.

Another crucial element in the onset and treatment of diverticulitis is diet. It is believed that a low-fiber diet has a significant role in the development of diverticula because it can cause constipation and elevated colonic pressure. Additional dietary variables that could raise the chance of diverticulitis include eating a lot of processed food, red meat, and refined carbohydrates.

Diverticulitis symptoms might vary according on how severe the illness is, but they typically include:

1. Pain in the abdomen, typically on the lower left side
2. Gas or bloating
3. Modifications in bowel habits, such diarrhea or constipation
4. Heat
5. Experiencing nausea and vomiting
6. Bleeding in the rectal area

More severe forms of diverticulitis can result in worsening symptoms as well as consequences including abscesses or perforations, which can be potentially fatal and necessitate emergency medical care.

Diverticulitis can be prevented by leading a healthy lifestyle and eating a balanced diet, which can help control symptoms in those who have already been diagnosed or lower the chance of getting the illness. Consuming a high-fiber diet full of fruits, vegetables, whole grains, and legumes is one of the most important preventive strategies. Fiber lowers the risk of diverticula formation by encouraging regular bowel movements and preventing constipation.

To keep your digestion in good working order and avoid constipation, drink lots of water to stay hydrated in addition to eating a high-fiber diet. Additionally, frequent exercise can support general digestive health and stool regularity. For those who have diverticulitis, avoiding particular foods like popcorn, seeds, almonds, and spicy meals may also be helpful in reducing symptoms.

Healthcare professionals may advise people with diverticulitis to adhere to a particular food plan in order to help control their symptoms and avoid flare-ups. When diverticulitis is acute, this diet usually consists of low-fiber meals; when symptoms subside, high-fiber foods are progressively added back in.

Conclusively, diverticulitis is a common gastrointestinal ailment that, if left untreated, can lead to discomfort and problems. People can lower their risk of having diverticulitis or effectively manage symptoms if they are already diagnosed by learning about the different varieties of the ailment, its origins, symptoms, and preventive actions like maintaining a good diet and lifestyle.

CHAPTER 1

FOODS TO EAT AND AVOID

𝓈ustaining a nutritious diet is essential for both treating diverticulitis and improving digestive health in general. Diverticulitis sufferers can lessen their symptoms, avoid flare-ups, and maintain optimal health by choosing their diets carefully. To support digestive health and well-being, we will examine what foods to eat and what to avoid on a diverticulitis diet in this chapter.

1. Foods to Eat

a. High-Fiber Foods: Eating foods high in fiber is a crucial part of a diverticulitis diet. Fiber can help avoid diverticula by promoting regular bowel movements, preventing constipation, and lowering colonic pressure. Fruits (apples, berries, pears), veggies (broccoli, carrots, spinach), whole grains (oats, brown rice, quinoa), and legumes (beans, lentils) are all good sources of fiber.

b. Foods High in Probiotics: Probiotics are good bacteria that promote gut health and aid in preserving a balanced population of microorganisms in the digestive system. Eating foods high in probiotics, such kefir, sauerkraut, kimchi, and yogurt, can aid in promoting digestive health and lowering colon inflammation.

c. Lean Protein Sources: By consuming less saturated fat, which can worsen the symptoms of diverticulitis, you can get the critical nutrients you need from lean protein sources including fish, chicken, tofu, and lentils.

d. Healthy Fats: To promote general digestive health and lessen inflammation in the body, choose healthy fats like those found in nuts, seeds, avocados, and olive oil.

e. Low-FODMAP Foods: Restricting certain kinds of carbohydrates that can aggravate digestive symptoms by eating a low-FODMAP diet may be beneficial for some people with diverticulitis. Rice, oats, some fruits (bananas, blueberries), and vegetables (bell peppers, zucchini) are examples of low-FODMAP foods.

2. Foods to Avoid:

a. High-Fat Foods: Steer clear of high-fat foods such processed meats, fried foods, and full-fat dairy items to help lower colon inflammation and stop diverticulitis symptoms from getting worse.

b. Spicy Foods: Consuming spicy food might aggravate the digestive system and exacerbate diverticulitis symptoms in some people. Preventing pain can be achieved by limiting or eliminating spicy foods like salsa, chili powder, and hot peppers.

c. Nuts and Seeds: Although it's debatable if these foods contribute to diverticulitis flare-ups, some medical professionals advise against eating them if symptoms are triggered or during acute episodes. Small amounts of seeds and nuts may be progressively reintroduced if well tolerated.

d. Popcorn: A high-fiber snack that might be challenging to digest and irritate the colon in many diverticulitis sufferers. Popcorn should be avoided or eaten in moderation, according to general recommendations.

e. Processed Foods: Foods heavy in chemicals, preservatives, and refined sugars can damage gut flora and exacerbate diverticulitis symptoms. Whenever possible, choose whole, minimally processed foods.

Conclusively, people with diverticulitis can effectively manage their condition and promote optimal digestive health by adhering to a balanced diet that includes high-fiber foods, probiotic-rich foods, lean proteins, healthy fats, and low-FODMAP options while avoiding high-fat foods, spicy foods, seeds and nuts, popcorn, and processed foods. Diverticulitis sufferers can improve their general health and lower their chance of flare-ups and other consequences from this common digestive ailment by choosing educated eating choices.

Benefits of following a Diverticulitis Diet

Seniors should pay special attention to their diet when it comes to diverticulitis disease since they are more vulnerable to digestive problems and may experience consequences from the disease. The main advantages of a diverticulitis diet for elderly people are as follows:

1. **Prevention of Flare-ups:** Elderly people can lessen the chance of flare-ups, which can result in bothersome symptoms such as

diarrhea, constipation, bloating, and abdominal discomfort, by adhering to a diverticulitis disease diet. High-fiber diets can encourage regular bowel movements and lower the risk of colon inflammation.

2. Symptom Management: Seniors who have diverticulitis may have symptoms like flatulence, cramps, and altered bowel patterns. Seniors can effectively control symptoms and enhance their overall quality of life by adopting a diet that is friendly on their digestive system.

3. Maintenance of Gut Health: Seniors with diverticulitis disease can benefit from a diet rich in foods strong in fiber, probiotics, lean proteins, and healthy fats. Seniors can improve their digestive health and lower their risk of complications from diverticulitis by encouraging a healthy balance of bacteria in the stomach and lowering inflammation in the colon

4. Preventing Complications: Seniors who have diverticulitis are more likely to experience complications such fistulas, abscesses, and perforations. Seniors can lessen their chance of developing these dangerous consequences by adhering to a diverticulitis illness diet that emphasizes lowering inflammation and boosting digestive health.

5. Nutritional Support: As seniors get older, their dietary requirements may alter, and they might need particular nutrients to maintain their general health and wellbeing. An array of nutrient-dense meals can give seniors with diverticulitis disease the vitamins, minerals, and antioxidants they need to stay healthy and active.

6. Weight Management: A diverticulitis diet may be beneficial for senior citizens with the illness in order to help them control their weight. Seniors can support weight management goals and lower their risk of obesity-related health concerns by eating a balanced diet high in fiber and low in saturated fats.

To sum up, seniors with diverticulitis disease can benefit greatly from adhering to a diet that promotes gut health, prevents complications, manages symptoms, prevents flare-ups, provides nutritional support, and helps them manage their weight. Seniors with diverticulitis can enhance their digestive health and general well-being as they age by practicing healthy eating habits and making educated food choices.

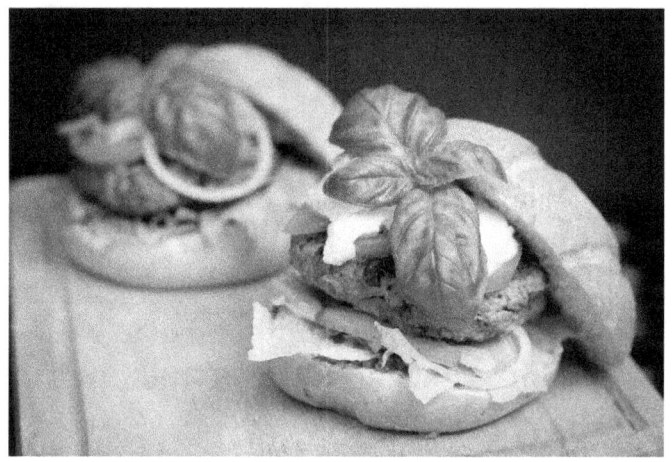

CHAPTER 2

HOW TO FOLLOW A DIVERTICULITIS DIET

A diverticulitis illness diet entails eating a certain way to help control symptoms, stop flare-ups, and maintain good digestive health. This is a thorough tutorial on how to adhere to a diet for diverticulitis:

1. Increase Fiber Intake: Eating a diet high enough in fiber is essential for treating diverticulitis. Foods high in fiber can help avoid constipation, encourage regular bowel movements, and lessen colon inflammation. Make it a goal to eat a lot of fruits, veggies, whole grains, legumes, and nuts every day.

2. Remain Hydrated: When adhering to a diverticulitis diet, it is imperative to consume copious amounts of water.

Maintaining adequate water lowers the likelihood of constipation by softening feces and making it easier to pass. Drink eight to ten glasses of water a day minimum, and stay away from alcohol and sugary drinks as these might worsen stomach problems.

3. **Limit Foods that may exacerbate Symptoms:** Some foods have the potential to exacerbate diverticulitis symptoms or cause flare-ups. These consist of foods that are spicy, heavy in fat, processed, contain red meat, dairy, and caffeine. Keep an eye on how your body responds to various foods and steer clear of any that seem to make you uncomfortable.

4. **Eat Foods High in Probiotics:** Probiotics are good bacteria that can support the gut microbiome's ability to remain in a balanced state. Consume foods high in probiotics, such as kefir, yogurt, sauerkraut, kimchi, and kombucha, to aid with digestion and lessen colon inflammation.

5. Select Lean Proteins: Go for lean protein sources including fish, eggs, chicken, and tofu. Compared to processed or fatty meats, these protein sources are less prone to cause digestive problems and are easier to digest.

6. Cook Foods Softly: Cooking food until it's soft and readily digestible may be beneficial during diverticulitis flare-ups or symptoms. Foods that are baked, boiled, or steamed can help break down fibers and be kinder to the digestive tract.

7. Eat Regular Meals: Making eating regular meals a habit will ease digestive discomfort and help control bowel movements. Instead of eating big meals that could tax the digestive system, try to eat modest, regular meals throughout the day.

8. Speak with a Dietitian: If you need help creating a diet plan for diverticulitis that suits your specific needs, think about speaking with a qualified dietitian. Based on your preferences, dietary constraints, and current state of health, a nutritionist can make tailored suggestions.

You may effectively manage symptoms of diverticulitis, lower the risk of flare-ups, and improve overall digestive health by adhering to these suggestions and making educated food choices. When making dietary adjustments, keep in mind that persistence and patience are essential, and it could take some time to notice benefits in your health.

SHOPPING INGREDIENTS

1. **Whole Grains:** To enhance your consumption of fiber, choose whole grains for your bread, pasta, brown rice, quinoa, and oats.

2. Fresh Fruits: Because they are high in fiber and nutrients, a range of fruits,

including bananas, berries, oranges, pears, and apples, should be chosen.

3. Vegetables: For their high fiber and vitamin content, stock up on bell peppers, sweet potatoes, broccoli, carrots, and leafy greens.

4. Legumes: Add beans, lentils, chickpeas, and peas to increase your intake of protein and fiber.

5. Nuts and Seeds: Eat unsalted walnuts, almonds, and flaxseeds for fiber and healthy fats, as well as chia, flax, and pumpkin seeds for seeds.

6. Low-Fat Dairy: For probiotics and to help maintain bone health, choose low-fat yogurt, milk, and cheese.

7. Lean Proteins: For protein that is low in fat, choose lean fowl, such as chicken or turkey, fish, such as salmon or tuna, tofu, and eggs.

8. Herbs and Spices: To add flavor without adding more salt, stock up on herbs and spices like oregano, ginger, garlic, turmeric, and basil.

9. Healthy Oils: To get healthy fats, use coconut, avocado, or olive oil in salad dressings and cooking.

10. Probiotic Foods: To improve gut health, think about including fermented foods like kefir, yogurt, sauerkraut, kimchi, and kombucha.

11. Natural Sweeteners: Rather than refined sugars, use natural sweeteners like stevia, honey, or maple syrup.

12. Whole Grain Crackers: For a snack that is easy on the stomach, go for rice cakes or whole grain crackers.

13. Canned Beans: Keep canned beans, such as kidney beans, chickpeas, or black beans, on hand for simple and quick meal additions.

14. Low-Sodium Broth: For easier-to-digest soups and stews, use low-sodium vegetable or chicken broth.

15. Nut Butter: Almond butter or peanut butter work well as a fruit and vegetable dip or as a spread for toast.

16. Coconut Water: Rich in electrolytes and a delicious beverage alternative, coconut water will help you stay hydrated.

17. Ingredients for Smoothies: Stock up on frozen fruits, such as spinach and berries, to make high-fiber smoothies with milk or yogurt.

18. Canned Fish: Add canned salmon or tuna for an easy way to get protein and omega-3 fatty acids.

19. Whole Grain Tortillas: To create a balanced dinner, use whole grain tortillas to make wraps with lean protein, veggies, and hummus.

20. **Green Tea:** Indulge in this antioxidant-rich, hydrating tea, which may also help with digestive health.

You may prepare balanced meals that support digestive health, lower inflammation, and enhance general well-being by adding these healthy shopping ingredients to your diet if you have diverticulitis disease. Never forget to pay attention to your body's needs and modify your diet according to how certain foods impact your symptoms.

Diverticulitis Disease Complications

Diverticulitis illness can have a number of consequences if the proper diet isn't followed. These side effects might be anything from little pain to serious medical problems. If the recommended diet is not followed, diverticulitis illness may result in the following possible complications:

1. Increased Inflammation: A low-fiber diet can aggravate the symptoms of diverticulitis and perhaps trigger flare-ups by increasing colon inflammation.

2. Persistent Symptoms: Digestion-related symptoms including cramping, bloating, constipation, diarrhea, and stomach discomfort can become chronic and persistent in the absence of a healthy diet.

3. Increasing Risk of Diverticular Bleeding: A low fiber diet can cause constipation and straining during bowel movements, which raises the possibility of diverticular bleeding, a potentially dangerous condition that has to be treated by a doctor.

4. **Risk of Perforation:** If severe diverticulitis is left untreated, it may develop in abscesses or perforations in the colon wall. If these injuries are not treated very once, they may cause sepsis or other dangerous infections.

5. **blockage:** A low-fiber diet may be a contributing factor in the development of bowel blockage or fecal impaction, which may necessitate surgery and cause excruciating stomach discomfort and bloating.

6. **Nutritional Deficiencies:** The immune system and general health can be weakened by a diet deficient in vital nutrients from fruits, vegetables, whole grains, and lean meats.

7. Increased Risk of Colon Cancer: If dietary modifications and medical care are not implemented to successfully control chronic inflammation and recurring episodes of diverticulitis, there may be a gradual rise in the risk of colon cancer.

8. Medication-related Complications: If dietary measures are insufficient to control diverticulitis symptoms, prescription drugs such antibiotics or analgesics may be necessary. These drugs come with dangers and side effects of their own when taken improperly.

In order to create a customized food plan that supports digestive health, lowers inflammation, and avoids problems, people with diverticulitis illness must collaborate closely with healthcare professionals, such as gastroenterologists and dietitians. People may assist in controlling their illness and lower their risk of complications from diverticulitis disease by eating a diet high in fiber, water, and nutrient-dense meals and avoiding trigger foods such as processed foods, red meat, and high-fat products.

CHAPTER 1

MEAL PLANNING

As it helps guarantee that they are consuming a balanced diet that promotes digestive health and lowers the risk of flare-ups and problems, meal planning is essential for people with diverticulitis. Meal planning has the following advantages for effective management, summarized here:

1. Consume Foods High in Fiber: Make an effort to include foods high in fiber in your meals, such as fruits, vegetables, whole grains, legumes, and nuts. Colon inflammation is decreased, constipation is avoided, and regular bowel movements are encouraged by fiber.

2. Keep Yourself Hydrated: Throughout the day, sip on lots of water to maintain a healthy digestive tract and avoid dehydration, which can exacerbate symptoms of diverticulitis.

3. Tiny, Frequent Meals: Rather than consuming big, heavy meals throughout the day, choose smaller, more frequent meals. By doing so, you may be able to avoid the diverticulitis-related bloating, gas, and belly pain.

4. Lean Protein sources: To maintain general nutrition and muscle function without aggravating symptoms of diverticulitis, incorporate lean protein sources such as fish, eggs, tofu, and chicken into your meals.

5. Steer Clear of Trigger meals: Red meat, processed meals, caffeine, alcohol, spicy foods, and high-fat foods are examples of foods that might exacerbate symptoms of diverticulitis. Determine which foods to avoid.

6. Cooking Techniques: To lessen the chance of escalating digestive problems, consider using moderate cooking techniques like steaming, baking, grilling, or boiling rather than frying or deep-frying.

7. Probiotic-Rich Foods: To support a healthy gut microbiota and enhance digestion, include probiotic-rich foods like yogurt, kefir, sauerkraut, and kombucha in your diet.

8. Speak with a Dietitian: Prepare a customized meal plan that satisfies your specific dietary requirements and successfully treats the symptoms of diverticulitis by working with a qualified dietitian or healthcare professional.

Benefits of Proper Meal Planning

1. Managing Symptoms: By supporting digestive health and lowering colonic inflammation, a well-planned diet can help relieve diverticulitis symptoms including diarrhea, bloating, constipation, and abdominal discomfort.

2. Avoidance of Flare-Ups: People can lessen their chance of developing problems from diverticulitis that may need medical attention by eating a well-balanced, nutrient- and fiber-rich diet.

3. Better Nutrition: By arranging meals, people with diverticulitis may make sure they are obtaining the nutrients they need from a range of food sources, which promotes immune system and general health.

4. Weight management: People may lessen their overall health and digestive system by following a well-planned diet that helps them maintain a healthy weight or, if required, lose weight.

5. Better Quality of Life: Diverticulitis patients who plan their meals well can enjoy a greater range of tasty, filling foods while efficiently controlling their condition, which enhances their quality of life.

Better symptom management, a lower chance of complications, and better overall health outcomes are all possible for people with diverticulitis illness who implement these meal planning techniques into their daily routine. To create a customized meal plan that satisfies dietary requirements and promotes the best possible management of diverticulitis, input from dietitians and healthcare professionals is crucial.

SIMPLE MEAL PLAN

This diet plan emphasizes low-fat, high-fiber meals to help maintain digestive health and stave off flare-ups:

First Day:

Greek yogurt with berries and chia seeds for breakfast; quinoa salad with grilled chicken and mixed vegetables for lunch; baked salmon with steamed asparagus and quinoa for dinner; and carrot sticks with hummus for a snack.

Day Two:

- Oatmeal with almonds and sliced bananas for breakfast
Lunch would be lentil soup paired with whole grain bread. Dinner would be

marinara sauced turkey meatballs over zucchini noodles.

- Snack: Almond butter on apple slices

Day Three:

Breakfast consists of whole grain toast and scrambled eggs with spinach. Lunch is a mixed green salad with grilled shrimp and avocado.

Dinner will be stir-fried tofu and vegetables over brown rice. For a snack, have Greek yogurt with honey and walnuts.

Day Four:

- Smoothie for breakfast made with almond milk, banana, spinach, and chia seeds

- Carrot sticks on the side with a turkey and avocado wrap for lunch
Supper is baked chicken breast paired with green beans and roasted sweet potatoes.
- Snack: Almond butter-topped rice cakes

Day Five:

- Lunch: Feta cheese, cucumbers, tomatoes, and chickpea salad
- Breakfast: Whole grain cereal with almond milk and sliced strawberries
- Fish tacos on the grill with salsa and cabbage slaw for dinner
- Snack: Dried fruit and mixed nuts

Day Six:

- Quinoa and black bean bowl with salsa and avocado for lunch; - Whole grain toast with avocado and poached eggs for breakfast

Dinner is baked turkey breast paired with quinoa and roasted Brussels sprouts. Snack is peanut butter-topped celery sticks.

Day Seven:

- Cottage cheese with sunflower seeds and slices of pineapple for breakfast
- Lunch will be grilled chicken and a salad of spinach and strawberries.

Snack: Almonds and berries; dinner is lentil curry over brown rice and steamed broccoli.

Always stay hydrated, steer clear of trigger foods, and pay attention to your body's cues. Adapt meal compositions and portion proportions to your specific requirements and tastes. Before making any major dietary changes, speak with a doctor or dietician to be sure they meet your unique health needs.

CHAPTER 4

BREAKFAST RECIPES

1. Yogurt Parfait with Blueberries and Almonds Ingredients:

– 1/2 cup Greek yogurt with reduced fat
One-fourth cup of raw blueberries
- One tablespoon of almonds, sliced
- One tablespoon of honey

Instructions: 1. Arrange the yogurt, almonds, and blueberries in a bowl or glass.
2. Pour honey over the top.
3. In only five minutes, savor this meal that's high in protein and fiber.

Nutritious Value: 250 Calories, 12g Protein, 4g Fiber

2. *Breakfast Bowl with Quinoa*

Ingredients: - 1/4 cup chopped walnuts
- 1/2 cup cooked quinoa
- 1/4 cup of apple dice
- One spoonful of maple syrup
A hint of cinnamon

Guidelines:
1. In a bowl, combine quinoa, apples, walnuts, maple syrup, and cinnamon.
2. Warm in the microwave for one minute.
3. In less than ten minutes, this substantial meal is ready.

Nutritional Value: 300 Calories, 8g Protein, and 6g Fiber

3. Berries and Chia Seed Oatmeal

Components:

One spoonful of chia seeds and half a cup of rolled oats

- 1/4 cup of berry mixture (blueberries, raspberries, and strawberries)
- One tablespoon of honey

Directions: 1. Prepare the oats per the directions on the package.

2. Add the chia seeds and sprinkle the mixed berries over top.

3. For more sweetness, drizzle honey over the top.

Nutritional Value: 280 Calories, 7g Protein, and 8g Fiber

4. Egg Scramble with Spinach and Feta

Ingredients:

- Two eggs
- 1/4 cup finely chopped spinach – 2 tablespoons of feta cheese crumbles

To taste, add salt and pepper.

Directions: 1. In a bowl, beat eggs and season with pepper and salt.

2. Use a nonstick skillet over medium heat to cook eggs.

3. Stir in feta cheese and spinach and simmer until eggs are fully cooked.

Nutritional Value: 280 Calories, 15g Protein, and 2g Fiber

5. Ingredients for Banana Almond Butter Toast:

One whole grain slice and one spoonful of almond butter

- Half a banana, cut

1. Toast the bread until it turns golden brown.
2. Arrange banana slices in a layer on top of the almond butter.
3. Savor this easy yet filling breakfast choice.

Nutritional Value: 220 calories, 6g of protein, and 4g of fiber

6. Pineapple and Cottage Cheese Bowl
Ingredients:

Half a cup of reduced-fat cottage cheese; half a cup of chopped pineapple; one tablespoon of shredded coconut

Directions: 1. In a bowl, combine cottage cheese and pineapple.

2. For extra taste, top with shredded coconut.

3. It takes just minutes to prepare this meal with a tropical flair.

Nutritional Value: 200 Calories, 15g Protein, and 2g Fiber

7. Smoked salmon on avocado toast

Components:

- 1 slice of whole grain bread – 1/4 mashed avocado
- Two smoked salmon slices
- Dill and lemon juice as garnish

1. Toast the bread until it becomes crispy.
2. Top with mashed avocado.
3. Arrange the slices of smoked salmon and garnish with dill and lemon juice.

Value for Nutrition: 250 Calories, 12g Protein, 5g Fiber

These nutritious breakfast recipes are not only delicious but also a great way to help elders with diverticulitis symptoms.

LUNCH RECIPES

1. Quinoa salad and grilled chicken

Ingredients: - 1 cup cooked quinoa - 1/2 cup grilled chicken breast, sliced - 4 ounces of mixed greens
- 1/4 cup chopped cucumber; - 1/4 cup cherry tomatoes; - 2 teaspoons balsamic vinaigrette

Guidelines:
1. Combine the quinoa, cucumber, cherry tomatoes, mixed greens, and grilled chicken in a bowl.
2. Add a balsamic vinaigrette drizzle and mix well.
3. In less than 15 minutes, savor this salad that is high in protein and fiber.

2. Soup with Lentils and Veggies

Components:
- 1/2 cup of lentils, dried
- One chopped carrot; - One chopped celery stalk; - Half a chopped onion
- 2 cups vegetable broth with minimal sodium - 1 teaspoon dried thyme

Guidelines:

After giving the lentils a good rinse, add the diced veggies, vegetable broth, and thyme to a pot.

2. Once the lentils are soft, bring to a boil, lower the heat, and simmer for 20 to 25 minutes.

3. It takes less than 30 minutes to prepare this filling and healthy soup.

3. Ingredients for the Turkey and Avocado Wrap:

One whole wheat tortilla and three ounces of sliced turkey breast
- 1/4 mashed avocado
1/4 cup of chopped lettuce
- 1/4 cup of bell peppers, chopped

1. Spread mashed avocado on top of the tortilla after it has been laid out.
2. Arrange the diced bell peppers, shredded lettuce, and turkey slices in layers.
3. For a quick and simple lunch alternative, roll up the wrap and cut in two.

4. Ingredients for the Quinoa and Salmon Bowl:

1/4 cup steaming broccoli florets, 1/4 cup sliced bell peppers, and 4 ounces of grilled fish fillet

Slicing lemons for decoration

Guidelines:

1. Arrange a bed of quinoa, top with sliced bell peppers and steam-broccoli. Place the grilled salmon on top.
2. To add more flavor, squeeze some fresh lemon juice over the bowl.
3. You can whip up this nutrient-dense meal in less than 20 minutes.

5. Stir-fried Vegetables and Chickpeas

Ingredients: - 1 cup mixed stir - 1/2 cup washed and drained canned chickpeas-fry veggies (carrots, snap peas, and bell peppers) -use two teaspoons of low-sodium soy sauce

A tsp of sesame oil

Guidelines:

1. Add mixed veggies and chickpeas to a skillet with hot sesame oil.
2. After the vegetables are crisp-tender, add the soy sauce and stir-fry for one more minute.
3. For a filling supper, serve this high-fiber stir-fry over brown rice.

6. Grilled shrimp in a Greek salad

Components:
- 1 cup mixed greens - 4 ounces grilled shrimp
- 1/4 cup chopped cherry tomatoes - 2 tablespoons feta cheese crumbles
- One tablespoon of olive oil

Guidelines:
1. In a bowl, mix together feta cheese, cherry tomatoes, mixed greens, and grilled shrimp.
2. Coat with a light drizzle of olive oil and toss to coat.
3. A light and revitalizing lunch choice is this salad with Mediterranean influences.

7. Vegetable and Turkey Skewers

Components:
- 4 ounces of diced turkey breast - 1/2 sliced zucchini
- Half a bell pepper, chopped
- One tablespoon of olive oil
- To taste, add salt, pepper, and garlic powder.

Guidelines:
1. Attach bell pepper chunks, zucchini slices, and turkey cubes to skewers.
2. Add a light olive oil brushing and sprinkle with garlic powder, salt, and pepper.
3. Cook the turkey and veggies on the skewers under the grill or in the oven until they are soft.

These lunch recipes are made to offer seniors who suffer from diverticulitis wholesome, simple-to-make, and mild options for their digestive systems.

DINNER RECIPES

1. Steamed asparagus and baked salmon with quinoa Ingredients:

- 1/2 cup cooked quinoa - 1 cup asparagus spears - 1 tablespoon olive oil
- 6 ounces of salmon fillet
- Slices of lemon as a garnish

Guidelines:
1. Set oven temperature to 200°C/400°F.
2. Transfer the salmon to a baking sheet, brush with olive oil, and sprinkle with salt and pepper to taste.
3. Bake the salmon for 15 to 20 minutes, or until it is cooked through.

4. Until tender, steam asparagus for five to seven minutes.

5. Present the cooked salmon atop quinoa, accompanied by steaming asparagus. Add slices of lemon as garnish.

2. *Brown rice stir-fried with turkey and vegetables*

Components:

- One cup of mixed stir-fried vegetables (carrots, broccoli, and bell peppers) - Two tablespoons of low-sodium soy sauce

- One cup of cooked brown rice - One tablespoon of sesame oil

Guidelines:

1. Cook the ground turkey in a skillet until browned.

2. Stir-fry the mixed vegetables until they are crisp-tender.
3. Add a little sesame oil and soy sauce, then simmer for one more minute.
4. For a well-balanced dinner option, serve brown rice with a stir-fried turkey and vegetables.

3. Black bean and Quinoa Stuffed Bell Peppers

Ingredients include one cup cooked quinoa, one can (15 oz) rinsed and drained black beans, and half a cup chopped and seeded bell peppers.
– 1/4 cup salsa

Guidelines:
1. Set oven temperature to 190°C/375°F.
2. Combine the quinoa, salsa, black beans, and corn in a bowl.

3. Once the bell peppers are soft, stuff the halves with the quinoa mixture and bake for 20 to 25 minutes.
4. Savor this filling dinner option of stuffed bell peppers, which are high in fiber.

4. Quinoa Pilaf with Vegetable and Chicken Skewers

Components:
- Eight ounces of diced chicken breast - One sliced zucchini - One chopped bell pepper
- One tablespoon of olive oil
- To taste, add salt, pepper, and garlic powder.
– 1/2 cup of quinoa, cooked

Guidelines:
1. Thread bits of bell pepper, zucchini, and chicken cubes onto skewers.

2. Add a light olive oil brushing and sprinkle with garlic powder, salt, and pepper.

3. Cook the chicken and veggies on the grill or in the oven until they are soft.

4. For a meal full of protein, serve the skewers over quinoa pilaf.

5. Salad of mixed greens and lentil soup

Ingredients:-Dried lentils, 1/2 cup
- One chopped carrot; - One chopped celery stalk; - Half a chopped onion
- One teaspoon of dried thyme - Two cups of low-sodium vegetable broth - Mixed greens for salad

1. Wash the lentils well and put them in a pot with chopped veggies, vegetable stock, and thyme.

2. Once the lentils are soft, bring to a boil, lower the heat, and simmer for 20 to 25 minutes.
3. For a well-balanced supper, serve lentil soup alongside a mixed green salad.

6. *Quinoa-Veggie Stir-Fry with Shrimp*
Ingredients: - One cup mixed stir - Six ounces of peeled and deveined shrimp-sauté veggies (bell peppers, mushrooms, and snap peas) -use two tablespoons of low-sodium soy sauce
1-Tbsp sesame oil - 1/2 cup quinoa that has cooked

Guidelines:
1. Add shrimp and mixed veggies to a skillet with heated sesame oil.
2. Stir-fry the veggies and shrimp until they are crisp-tender and pink.

3. Add a soy sauce drizzle and simmer for a minute more.
4. For a tasty supper alternative, serve stir-fried shrimp and vegetables over quinoa.

7. Feta Cheese with Greek Chicken Salad

Components:
- 6 ounces of sliced grilled chicken breast - 1 cup of mixed greens
- 1/4 cup chopped cherry tomatoes - 2 tablespoons feta cheese crumbles - 1 tablespoon olive oil
- A dressing of lemon juice

Guidelines:
1. In a bowl, mix together feta cheese, cherry tomatoes, mixed greens, and grilled chicken.

2. As a dressing, drizzle with olive oil and lemon juice.

3. For a light and refreshing supper option, try this chicken salad with Mediterranean influences.

These suppertime recipes provide seniors with diverticulitis pleasant, easy-to-prepare, and healthy options that are also mild on the digestive tract.

SNACKS RECIPES

1. Berries and almonds with a Greek yogurt parfait

Components: - Half a cup of Greek yogurt

- 1/4 cup of mixed berries, including strawberries and blueberries; - 2 teaspoons of almond slices

Guidelines:

1. Arrange Greek yogurt, sliced almonds, and mixed berries in a bowl or glass.

2. Savor this fiber- and protein-rich parfait as a filling after-meal.

2. *Veggie and Hummus Platter*

Components:

- 1/4 cup hummus
- One little cucumber, cut
- One carrot, thinly sliced
- One-fourth cup cherry tomatoes

Guidelines:

1. Arrange cherry tomatoes, carrot sticks, cucumber slices, and hummus on a platter.

2. Dip the vegetables in hummus to make a wholesome and crispy snack.

3. Rice Cake with Slices of Avocado and Tomato

Ingredients: - 1/4 mashed avocado - 1 rice cake

- Two tomato slices

Directions: 1. Top a rice cake with tomato pieces after spreading mashed avocado on it.

2. The fiber and healthy fats in this easy and light snack.

4. Pineapple Chunks with Cottage Cheese

Components:

- 1/2 cup of reduced-fat cottage cheese
- 1/2 cup of chunked pineapple

Instructions: 1. In a bowl, mix together cottage cheese and slices of pineapple.

2. Savor this food that is high in protein and has a hint of sweetness.

5. On whole grain crackers, almond butter

Components:
- Two teaspoons of almond butter - Two whole grain crackers

Directions: 1. For a crisp and filling snack, spread almond butter on whole grain crackers.
2. The combo provides healthful fats and a decent source of protein.

6. Chia Seed Pudding with Mixed Berries -

Add 2 teaspoons of chia seeds to the mixture.

- 1/2 cup almond milk without sugar - 1/4 cup mixed berries (blackberries and raspberries)

Guidelines:

1. To thicken, combine chia seeds and almond milk in a bowl and refrigerate for at least 30 minutes.

2. For a pudding that is high in fiber and nutrients, sprinkle mixed berries on top.

7. Apple Slices with Cinnamon and Almond Butter

Ingredients: - One sliced apple
- Two tsp almond butter
- A dash of cinnamon

Directions: 1. Drizzle apple slices with almond butter and cinnamon.

2. The perfect balance of fiber, protein, and natural sweetness may be found in this tasty snack.

These ideas for delicious and easy-to-make snacks are great for anyone with diverticulitis, as they are light on the stomach.

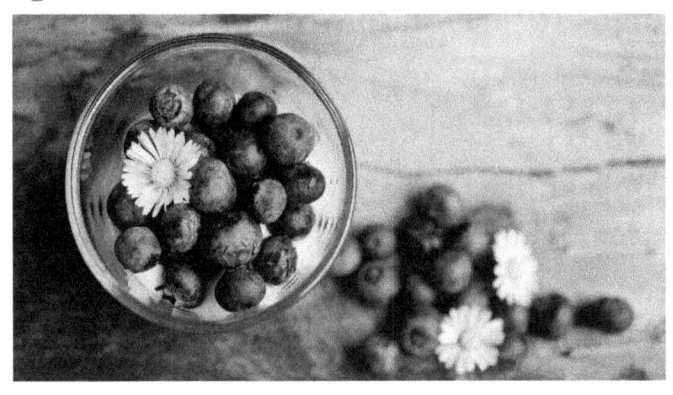

CONCLUSION

To sum up, this senior diverticulitis disease cookbook is a great tool for anyone dealing with the difficulties associated with the illness. Not only are the dishes tasty and nourishing, but they are also designed to support digestive health and general wellbeing. You can take proactive measures to control the symptoms of diverticulitis and enhance your quality of life by including these meals in your diet.

I invite you, my dear reader, to use this cookbook as a healing and empowering tool. Take these recipes as a roadmap to improved health and increased energy. Never forget that each meal you eat is an opportunity to help your digestive system and nourish your body.

Finally, I would like you to write a review of this cookbook so that you can share your ideas and experiences. Others dealing with diverticulitis-related difficulties may find inspiration and support in your comments. In the face of hardship, we may unite as a community and show support for one another. I appreciate you joining me on this gastronomic journey. Continue to be healthy, powerful, and to cook with love.

Wishing you Good Health

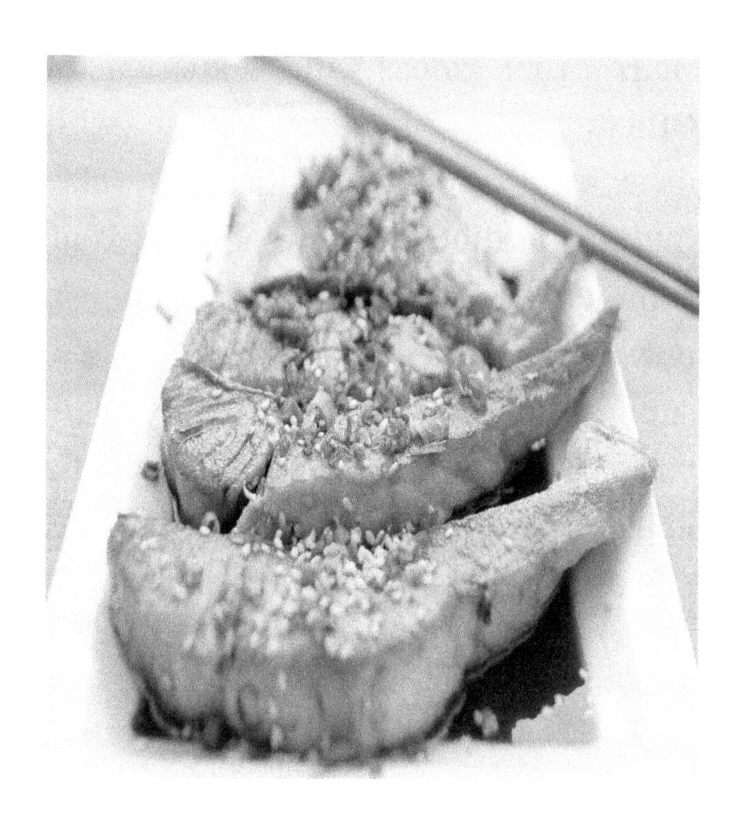

Printed in the USA
CPSIA information can be obtained
at www.ICGtesting.com
LVHW022253110924
790847LV00007B/168